THE ESSENTIAL HANDBOOK FOR APPLE CIDER VINEGAR

TIPS AND RECIPES FOR WEIGHT LOSS

AND IMPROVING YOUR HEALTH,

BEAUTY, AND HOME

By

EVELYN CARMICHAEL

Copyright © 2016

Evelyn Carmichael

INTRODUCTION

Like me, you've walked into the supermarket a zillion times. How many times have you gone down the condiment aisle and seen apple cider vinegar and wondered, "So what's the difference?" At first glance, the only difference is the brown color and it is not as clear as the one you are used to picking up. Little do most people know that apple cider vinegar is jam-packed with some amazing uses.

Well, perhaps this is the right moment you should be reading this handbook. In it you will discover the essential uses and benefits of apple cider vinegar. Find out how you can use this all natural product for your home, in your beauty regime, for your health, and help you lose weight! All this and it is a common product you have probably had sitting on a shelf in your pantry for years! Discover how organic apple cider vinegar can lower blood sugar levels and aid other health issues such as high cholesterol, coughs and colds and poor digestion. It also provides a boost for your ever-fighting immune system.

Evelyn Carmichael

This Essential Handbook guides you uses of Apple Cider Vinegar in four main categories- to lose weight, your health, your body and beauty routine, and for your home. We will dive into these categories and you will learn tidbits like this amazing product provides an alternative to chemically produced cosmetics and therefore a gentle ingredient for your skin care routine. Also, each section has recipes on how to use for the particular remedy. As to your food, check out the recipe chapter. Apple cider vinegar gives your soups zest and lifts your sauces and salads plus some innovative recipes you will definitely want to try. Furthermore, apple cider vinegar is never outdone by household cleaners. Read on to see how Apple Cider Vinegar is your alternative to a more natural, environmentally-friendly and pet-friendly solution for your home and garden.

The Essential Handbook for Apple Cider Vinegar

Evelyn Carmichael

The Essential Handbook for Apple Cider Vinegar

TABLE OF CONTENTS

Evelyn Carmichael

LEGAL NOTES

Evelyn Carmichael

CHAPTER 1. HOW IT ALL STARTED

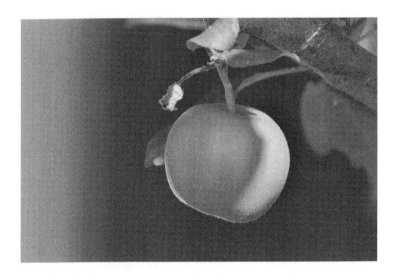

Never would you think that so lowly a product could have such powerful effects on everyday living. The product we are talking about here is apple cider vinegar, for short referred to also as ACV. Apple cider vinegar is not just a modern-day solution. It has its existence framed in history also. In 5000 B.C. the Babylonians fermented the date palm to produce wine. However, in the whole process a wine that was quite soured developed (by accident, that is) and they used it for pickling foods. The Egyptians of 3000 BC also produced something similar in their quest to make wine from barley. They used the vinegar as part of their medicinal folklore as traces of the substance has been found in their urns of that era.

It is Hippocrates however, the great physician whose name has been linked to the use of apple cider vinegar made from the fermentation of apples. Hippocrates prescribed the vinegar mixed with honey for a variety of ailments including coughs and colds. As a matter of fact, Hippocrates would use the substance to clean wounds also. Perhaps it is this important reason why the substance was used in both the US civil war and in World War 1 to treat the wounds of soldiers. Apple cider vinegar found favor elsewhere because the Japanese Samurai warriors drank it to enhance their strength and power while ancient Persians would dilute it to prevent fat from accumulating in their bodies. Many other instances of the use of apple cider vinegar in history in different parts of the world have been documented.

The benefits of ACV had become even more recognized with the publication of a folk medicine book by Dr. D. C. Javis in 1958. The doctor recommended ACV as a cure for many illnesses because:

- Of Its high potassium content.
- It was seen to be very effective when mixed with honey.
- It was a powerful fighting agent against destructive bacteria in the digestive tract.
- It aided digestion when it was taken with meals.

Apple cider vinegar is unlike the clear filtered vinegar that is more evident on your supermarket shelves. Instead, it has a brown juice colored concentration and is generally made from the juice of crushed apple or other fruit and herbs. Usually, the juice is left to ferment into an alcoholic state. Cultured bacteria is added to it which turns this alcoholic substance into acetic acid. Acetic acid is the active compound in ACV, giving it the appearance of wine. This in fact is what vinegar means in French, "sour wine".

Evelyn Carmichael

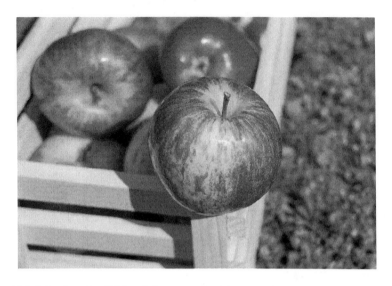

Which Apple Cider Vinegar to Use

Apple cider vinegar however makes all the difference when the culture of bacteria is allowed to remain in the vinegar. This is vinegar that is unfiltered or that does not go through the process of pasteurization. Apple cider vinegar in its raw unprocessed state is said to contain the "Mother" and has the appearance of a murky web-like substance. It is this version of vinegar that is so beneficial in many aspects of living. This is why it is so important to buy organic apple cider vinegar. The unfiltered organic version contains the "Mother".

The Essential Handbook for Apple Cider Vinegar

Evelyn Carmichael

CHAPTER 2. APPLE CIDER VINEGAR AND YOUR HEALTH

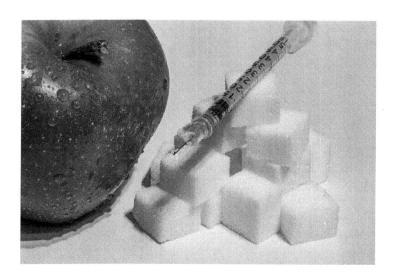

We are often reminded of the very old cliché "An apple a day, keeps the doctor away", an apt way to tell us of the importance of eating apples, or fruits, for that matter. This saying must have been coined because of the richness in nutrients found in apples. This is a wonder fruit as it acts on the body from two

Evelyn Carmichael

perspectives. One, the fruit is found to be moderately high in potassium which keeps your soft body tissues such as the muscles and arteries strong. This is why apples are such good anti-aging agent. On the other hand, apples are filled with calcium, that nutrient that maintains hard tissues such as your bones. For these reasons, ACV is considered high in the nutrients that come from the fruits that make it.

Help with Diabetes

While ACV is not a cure-all for illnesses, many people are able to attest to the benefits of the product in one way or another. In order to experience the true benefit, probably you should test it yourself. For example, ACV has been tested scientifically and found to reduce blood sugar levels. This is especially true in persons who have type 2 diabetes. Diabetes is a disease that occurs either because the body is resistant to the insulin it produces to control sugar in the blood, or it cannot produce the insulin to take care of the problem. Of course, if you have diabetes you well know you would be at great risk if you do not put a lid on the type of foods you eat, especially sugars. Apple Cider Vinegar has been shown to help reduce your blood sugar level, even when you haven't eaten exactly as you should. It has been found that just taking some ACV mixed with water improves the uptake of insulin in the body by between 19 – 34% especially when you have a meal high in carbohydrates. You would be surprised to know that two tablespoons of ACV taken before bedtime will cause your blood sugar to go down in the morning.

Help with High Cholesterol

High cholesterol levels in the body have been known to contribute heavily to heart disease and stroke. Furthermore, these diseases have been linked to high death rates. Although studies are limited, there is some scientific evidence that if you regularly ingest some ACV you would have a reduction in bad cholesterol. It is believed that the action of the antioxidant chlorogenic acid in ACV has much to do with preventing cholesterol deposits from crystalizing on the walls of your blood vessels, effectively lessening the deadly effects that can occur. A study that was done at Harvard University found that women who ate salads mixed with ACV had a reduced risk of heart disease than others who did not [2].

Help with Colds and Sinuses

What would many people give for a product that can relieve their sinus and cold symptoms? Many have been afflicted with sinus infections, sometimes seasonally, and there are those who will tell you it accompanies them throughout the year. Many will swear however that ACV does what regular medicine had not done for them. Some have gone to the point of ending their prescription medication. The potassium in ACV works to thin the mucus in the nasal passage while the acetic acid kills the germs that cause the problem to recur. Apple cider vinegar also has been used locally to ease and prevent the symptoms of the regular cold which causes such great misery on an average person of twice per year. A tablespoon of ACV will quickly dissolve the mucus and cause the nasal fluid to dry up. The solution also often takes care of a sore throat with just a gargle.

Help with Digestive Health Issues

Many people suffer from digestive problems, not to mention the very common acid reflux. This happens when the contents of the stomach flow back into the esophagus or food pipe. This can cause a real burning sensation and you get what is often called heart burn. Some persons also get this awful pain when they eat certain types of food. Apple cider vinegar has been found to provide tremendous relief from these digestive issues, especially when it is taken before a meal. A tablespoonful may be all you need to start eating your favorite foods that you had been avoiding.

Supports the Immune System

The immune system protects all other systems of the body against the invasion of harmful agents such as bacteria and viruses. The immune system itself however needs to be strengthened to carry out its work. Apple cider vinegar has long been used to provide this sort of boost to the immune system. There is the story that is often told of the thieves who survived the bubonic plague of the 1300s - 1700s in England because they drank a fermented vinegar brew made from herbs like rosemary, lavender and thyme. People in the villages and towns of England during the time of the bubonic plague also made stone crosses which they set up in the market places. The stone crosses were made with a depression which they filled with vinegar to drop coins in to kill the bacteria that caused the disease. This helped to stem the spread of the disease [3].

Evelyn Carmichael

CHAPTER 3. APPLE CIDER VINEGAR AND LIFESTYLE ISSUES

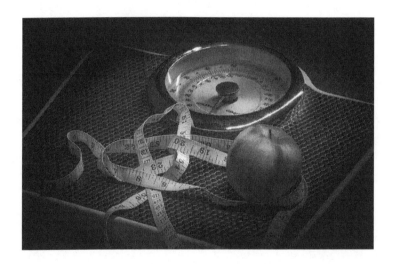

Help with Weight Loss

Many have struggled with weight issues and have tried different ways to lose the extra pounds. There are those of us also where weight is not a health issue, but for aesthetic reasons, we want to drop a few pounds. A combination of exercise and diet are the most effective ways to lose and maintain weight.

This is not a lifestyle however that is easy to maintain. Whether it is the temptation of the very high calorie foods that we are not supposed to eat, or not having the discipline to stretch and torture our bodies for 30 minutes every day, weight loss can be difficult. One thing is for certain, a little bit of ACV per day is never too difficult a discipline to maintain. What ACV does is to suppress your appetite so you feel full and at the same time boost your metabolism leading to weight loss. In addition, it prevents water retention. As mentioned before if blood glucose levels are improved by ACV, it will eventually translate into losing weight.

Help with Detoxification

Over time your body produces toxins as a result of processing all the foods and chemicals that we take in. A buildup of toxins cannot be beneficial to us but rather harms the body making you feel less energetic, unable to lose weight, creates mood swings, gaseous and bloated stomachs, headaches, fogginess of the brain, bad breath and body odors, spotty and itchy skin, indigestion and so forth. For these reasons, it is recommended you have a periodic detox to flush unhealthy substances from the body. You may sign up with a detox program and that is commendable. However, ACV is a good detoxifier in itself that aids in cleansing the liver and giving you more energy to do your daily activities. You can make it into a simple tea type of warm drink by adding a tablespoon of ACV mixed in a cup of warm water, a teaspoon of raw honey, and a squeeze of lemon juice.

Balances your pH Level

Your body needs a balance in pH level, that is, it should not be too acidic or alkaline. In fact, there should be a greater measure of alkalinity than acidity in the body. Apple cider vinegar is naturally alkaline and makes the body less acidic. This balance prevents bacteria and certain diseases from developing and gives you more energy. So instead of reaching for a bottle of energy drink to give you a punch in your daily activities, have a tablespoon of ACV in a glass of water. Some people use the mixture while they are having their exercise workout too to prevent a build-up of lactic acid which causes muscle cramps.

Evelyn Carmichael

CHAPTER 4. APPLE CIDER VINEGAR AS A BEAUTY PRODUCT

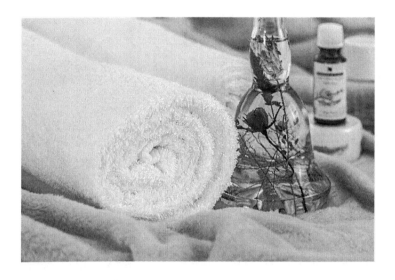

For the beauty conscious person, there is never a moment that you are not sniffing out the best products that can make your hair and skin shine with beauty and luster. Some persons however are more particular and would prefer natural products than chemically prepared ones to make the difference. You will think that the high acidity of ACV may be too harsh for beauty care. Well, you are ever so wrong as you will find it as gentle a product as any beauty care product at the cosmetic counter. ACV has long been used in cosmetic care and even in ancient Roman Empire, it was used to tone the skin. Cleopatra, famed beauty queen of ancient Egypt knew the value of the vinegar. The story is often told of how Cleopatra wagered with Marc Anthony that she could swallow a fortune in just one meal. Cleopatra is said to have dissolved a pearl in vinegar and drank it to prove she could.

For Beautiful Shiny Hair

If your hair is not getting that bounce and sheen that it should have, perhaps you can try some ACV in a rinse once per week. The acidity of ACV gives the hair a healthier look and leaves it soft and shiny. You will also discover that it is great in detangling the hair as it allows you to comb through more freely. In addition to providing a good pH balance for your scalp, it prevents products from building up on the hair. Instead of spending a fortune on clarifying or dandruff shampoo, try some ACV once a week. Apple cider vinegar can be used by itself or you may mix it with other products such as baking soda to treat your hair. Prepare a mixture of 1/3 cup vinegar to 4 cups water and use it to rinse the hair after shampooing. Then rinse the hair with water.

Use to Tone the Skin and Fade Blemishes

As with the hair, ACV balances the pH level of your skin to give it that healthy glow and feel. The nutrients in the product are also known to reduce aging. It is also used by some to treat acne and psoriasis. If you suffer from any of these problems, pour a solution of ACV and water on cotton swab and rub lightly on the skin for a deep clean or to remove blemishes.

Use as a Deodorant

Cosmetic deodorants can be harsh on especially sensitive skin. You may be one of those people who get a rash or bumps when you use them. ACV can be your alternative to allergic reactions to these types of products. Dilute a teaspoon of ACV in water and use a wash cloth to apply the solution under your arm. The beautiful thing is that it is absorbed and you do not need to worry about vinegar scent when it dries.

Removes Warts and Fades Skin Blemishes

Warts are unsightly skin blemishes some of us wish we did not have. They are often difficult to remove or hide unless you have them surgically removed. You can however treat some warts naturally with ACV by consistently applying a little of the solution to the area. After a while the growth will eventually fall off. Moles and bruises are also treatable with ACV. The product has anti-inflammatory effects and will fade the discoloration on the skin.

Molluscum contagiosum, a skin rash many children get, has also been shown to be treatable by ACV. Putting a cotton swap soaked in ACV on the affected area will often show results quickly and reduce irritation for your child without having to use steroid based creams. If your child is sensitive to the direct solution, you can dilute it by putting the ACV on a wet cotton ball or dilute with one part water prior to putting on the cotton.

Whitens Teeth and Freshens the Breath

You can smile again with confidence by using ACV to remove stains from your teeth. Rub the compound directly on the teeth or place a diluted amount in your mouth and swish it around for a minute or two. Brush your teeth as usual. Bacteria can build up at an alarming rate in orifices like the mouth causing offensive odors. This happens especially after having a meal and when you've eaten certain kinds of food that are more likely to cause bacteria to develop. Apple cider vinegar has been known to provide relief when it is used as a mouthwash as it helps in destroying the odor-causing bacteria. Just dilute and gargle.

Use as a Massage Treatment

If you are on your feet day in and day out or use your hands frequently throughout the day, ACV can be a great relief to your tired hands and feet. Place some of the liquid in your hands and rub on your hands and feet. Relax and do a good rub and enjoy the sensation it gives. You'll get a more soothing effect if you have someone to do it for you. As a bonus, if there is any trouble with smelly feet, ACV will take care of it.

Evelyn Carmichael

CHAPTER 5. APPLE CIDER VINEGAR AROUND THE HOME

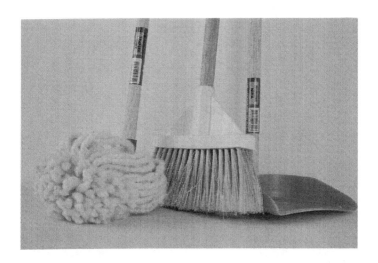

Use as a Cleaning Solution

Vinegar has been used in many households the world over as a cleaning agent. Its high acidic nature makes it an excellent cleaning solution used to cut grease and grime, destroy bacteria, and eliminate bacteria causing odors. This is a wonderful alternative to the number of chemicals we tend to use and toxins we unknowingly expose ourselves to. Apple cider vinegar may have that sour smell while using it. You need not worry however as the odor disappears when it dries. It will clean your kitchen surfaces and ovens. Just pour a little in the dishwasher and it acts as a detergent giving a sparkle to your dishes. You can also use it to clean windows, glasses and mirrors without leaving any streak. In the bathroom, it is the perfect disinfect. Just pour a little in the toilet and ACV freshens the air for you.

Use to discourage Fruit Flies

When Myna Warren had an invasion of fruit flies in her kitchen and bathroom, she did not know what was going on. Neither did her friends and work colleagues when she asked for their ideas in ridding the little pests that would not go away, but seemed to rather multiply in great numbers. She used copious amounts of store bought disinfectants and insect repellants. But the flies instead increased in numbers and with an indication they were not going anywhere soon. It was only when she took her dilemma to the Internet that she got information and a welcome relief from the fruit flies. There she discovered those little bugs can be an annoyance and very difficult to get rid of. Apple cider vinegar was found to be the perfect cure for them. Pour about ½ an inch of ACV in a cup or bottle. Add a bit of soap and cover the container with a piece of paper or plastic wrap. Use a rubber band to hold it in place around the mouth of the cup. Make holes in the cover and the vinegar will attract the flies and draw them in. You can also use this trap to catch larger bothersome flies around the home.

Use as a Weed Killer

One of the great benefits that can be had from ACV is its power to kill unwanted weeds in your garden. It is a wonderful alternative to commercial weedicides that are high in chemicals and that destroy the natural environment. Unlike these products, the acidity in ACV and its organic ingredients act against weeds, while providing a more effective way of building the soil it treats. Depending on the size of the area that you want to treat, mix about 2 liters of ACV with some salt and liquid detergent. Put in a spray bottle and pour on weeds without fear of chemical weed killers.

Use as a Flea and Tick Repellant

Dogs and cats are perpetually hounded (no pun intended) by fleas and ticks. If you are an animal lover you will almost always be seeking ways to combat the little critters. You are wise to the fact that if your pet is infected, you could be very soon! They can cause you serious skin irritation and all you get is frustration when your efforts are fruitless. Apple cider vinegar again comes to the rescue as an inexpensive alternative to chemicals that are often not effective. Here's how ACV works: Mix a solution of one part ACV with one part water. Use it to spray into your pet's coat or if you would rather, bathe the animal with the mixture. Spray around the house also. Do this for about a week and the fleas will disappear. For added effect, mix a few drops of ACV in your pets' drinking water. Only ensure that the vinegar used is the organic natural ACV.

The Essential Handbook for Apple Cider Vinegar

Evelyn Carmichael

CHAPTER 6. APPLE CIDER VINEGAR IN YOUR FOOD

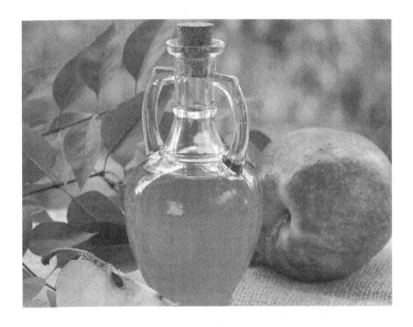

Wherever you go, a bottle of vinegar can be found in the food pantry of many households. Apple cider vinegar has been widely used in a variety of ways to add taste and nutritive value to food. Here are some ways you can add ACV to your diet.

In Soups

Soups are delightful and easy to make meals that even picky eaters often enjoy. You can use ACV to jazz up your soups for a great flavor. Only use in moderate proportions so it won't overpower the other ingredients. A tablespoon or two will do the trick. It also helps to brighten the colors in your soup.

In Sauces and Marinades

Almost every person has tried his or her hands at making a good sauce for your roast, barbecue or stew. Whether you'd rather make it yourself, or you prefer to pick up a bottle from the store shelf, vinegar is often a prominent ingredient in marinades. Nothing beats ACV in a good pot roast. To start with, add ACV to your favorite herbs and spices as a marinade for meats. It acts as a tenderizer for tough cuts of meat. Try using it to make a pickle for vegetables and herbs. Drizzle a little on sautéed or fried fish too and your family and friends will keep coming back for more.

Salad Dressings

Everyone knows that the best salad dressing is made with vinegar as the base ingredient. You can find dressings on the store shelves to reduce time in the kitchen. However, if you are like many of us and you are up to it, you only need to whisk in some ACV with olive oil and any of your other favorite ingredients such as garlic, honey and mustard. This will certainly make your vegetables, pasta or other salads come alive and taste great. The great thing about ACV is that it comes without the calories.

Juices

Generally, ACV can be had on its own to benefit from its healthy ingredients. However, if you feel that it may be a bit harsh to swallow, add it to juices for a great taste. In fact, you can make an ACV tonic by mixing it with fruit drinks and storing it for a few days in the fridge. An ACV berry tonic for example will delight you with color and flavor. Many people are now going for smoothies as a healthy alternative or addition to their diet. Smoothies can taste better with a little ACV added.

The Essential Handbook for Apple Cider Vinegar

Evelyn Carmichael

Chapter 7. Cooking with Apple Cider Vinegar

You may well be acquainted with your bottle of ACV as it sits on the shelf in your food cupboard. Yes, you know it is beneficial as a household cleaner and it cannot be left out of a marinade for your meats or to help build a good vinaigrette for salads. Apple cider vinegar may be one of the most unlikely of products you will consider for your menus. However, this chapter provides an opportunity to explore some ways you can incorporate ACV in your cooking for some of the most delicious meals for friends and families. Whether it is to make a refreshing punch, adding flavor to meats, or to present a scrumptious dessert, you'll find apple cider vinegar a very versatile ingredient. You can't beat a good apple cider vinegar glaze; the recipe is included below!

You can use the following drinks to get your daily dose of apple cider vinegar. Having these early in the morning is bound to give you that energy to bring you through the day. You will however find them very delicious to pair with your entrees.

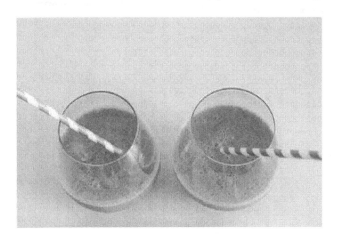

Pink Super Juice

Ingredients

1 ½ cups pink grapefruit juice

1 – 1 1/2 tbsp. Apple Cider Vinegar

2 tsp. raw honey

Method: Mix together all the ingredients in a glass. Chill and have it with your meal.

Evelyn Carmichael

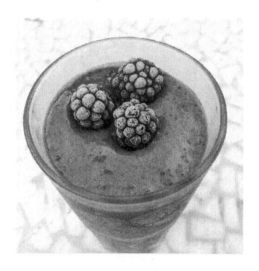

Smoothie

Ingredients

1cup of fruit (frozen berries, banana)

1 ½ tbsp. Apple Cider Vinegar

1 cup of Greek vanilla yogurt

Ice

Method: Mix in blender until all ingredients are smooth.

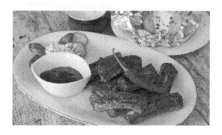

Apple Cider Vinegar Barbecue Sauce

Ingredients

2 c. ketchup

1/2 c. Apple sauce

1/2 c. apple cider

1/3 c. apple cider vinegar

1/4 c. Worcestershire sauce

2 tsp. Dijon mustard

3/4 tsp. garlic powder

1/2 tsp. onion powder

1 tsp. kosher salt

1/4 tsp. freshly ground pepper

Method: Stir together all the ingredients in a saucepan over medium heat. Let the sauce simmer for about 15 minutes until the flavors blend and it thickens slightly. Remove from the heat and let it cool. Pour into a tightly covered jar and you can use as desired in your burgers or on your meats.

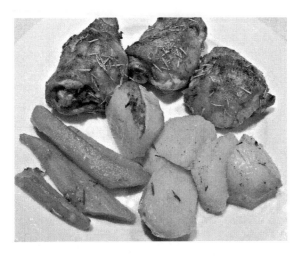

Maple Chicken and Carrots with ACV

Ingredients

4 chicken thighs with bone and skin on

kosher salt

Freshly ground black pepper

2 tbsp. extra-virgin olive oil

1/4 c. apple cider vinegar

3 cloves garlic, minced

1/4 c. maple syrup

2 tbsp. whole-grain mustard

1 tbsp. fresh thyme leaves

Evelyn Carmichael

Juice of 1/2 lemon

3 large carrots, peeled and sliced into 1/4"-thick
rounds

Method: Set your oven to heat at 425^0 F. Season
the chicken thighs with salt and pepper. Heat half the
oil in a large enough oven-safe skillet and sear the
chicken for 2 minutes on each side. Transfer the
chicken on to a plate when this is done.

Pour in the ACV in the skillet and use a wooden
spoon to scrape any bits left on the bottom of the
skillet. Throw in the garlic, maple syrup, mustard,
thyme, and lemon juice and bring to a boil. Place the
chicken back in the skillet and spoon the sauce over
it.

Mix the carrot with the remaining oil, salt and pepper
and place in the skillet around and between the
thighs. Bake for about 20 minutes or until chicken and
carrot are tender. Serve with the delicious pan sauce.

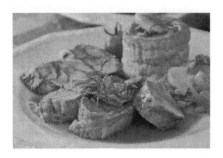

Apple Cider Vinegar Glazed Pork

Ingredients

1/2 c. apple cider

2 tbsp. apple cider vinegar

1 tbsp. whole-grain Dijon mustard

1 (1–1 1/2 lbs.) pork tenderloin

Kosher salt

Freshly ground black pepper

2 tsp. chopped fresh rosemary

3 tbsp. butter, divided

1 tbsp. extra-virgin olive oil

Method: Set your oven to 400⁰ F. Use a whisk to mix the cider, cider vinegar, and mustard. Remove any fat from the pork and season with the salt, pepper, and rosemary. Heat both butter and oil in an oven-safe skillet and sear the pork on each side until golden brown. Place the skillet with the pork into the oven and roast until the temperature of the meat reaches 140^0 F. (Test with a food thermometer).

Remove the pork to a plate. Add the vinegar sauce to the contents of the skillet and let simmer. Loosen the bits on the bottom with a wooden spoon. Return the pork to the skillet, baste with the sauce and cook for few minutes more until the sauce thickens.
Let the pork rest for a while then slice. Drizzle the sauce over the sliced meat and serve.

You can use this Apple Cider Vinegar Glaze on different meats. It would be delicious on turkey, chicken, or even fish.

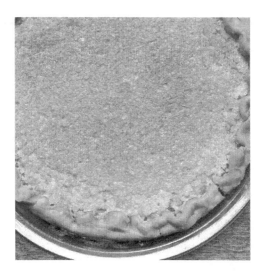

Apple Cider Vinegar Pie

Ingredients

4 large eggs

2 cups sugar

5 tbsps. corn starch

¼ teaspoon salt

1 ounce (2 tbsps.) apple cider vinegar

2 cups water

½ teaspoon vanilla extract

2 tbsps. butter, room temperature (optional)

Evelyn Carmichael

Pre-baked 9" pie crust, graham cracker or pastry

Method: Set your oven to 350^0 F. Combine eggs, sugar, cornstarch and salt and whisk well. Add the water and vinegar and whisk until the mixture is smooth. Cook the mixture over medium heat until it thickens to coat the back of a spoon. Remove from heat and mix in the vanilla extract and butter. Pour the mixture in a prepared pie crust. Then bake the pie for 15 – 18 minutes until it is set and barely jiggles when you move the pan. Let the pie cool and then place in refrigerator for at least 4 hours before serving.

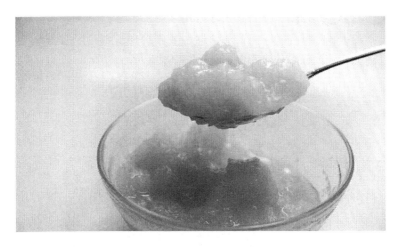

Chunky Apple Sauce

Ingredients

8 cups of chopped, peeled, tart apples

¼ c. Apple Cider Vinegar

½ c. packed brown sugar (or sugar substitute)

1 tsp cinnamon

1tsp vanilla

Directions

In large pot or Dutch oven, combine apples, brown sugar and cinnamon. Cover and cook over medium-

Evelyn Carmichael

low heat 30-40 minutes or until apples are tender, stirring occasionally. Remove from heat; stir in ACV and vanilla. Mash apples slightly if desired. Serve warm or cold. Yield: about 6 servings or 3-1/2 cups.

Variations

Mix 1 cup of fresh cranberries in with the apples to cook

Add raisins (approx. 1 cup) to make a chutney

Try various berries, pears, figs, or even nuts to make a wonderful side dish

The Essential Handbook for Apple Cider Vinegar

Evelyn Carmichael

CHAPTER 8. USING APPLE CIDER VINEGAR SAFELY

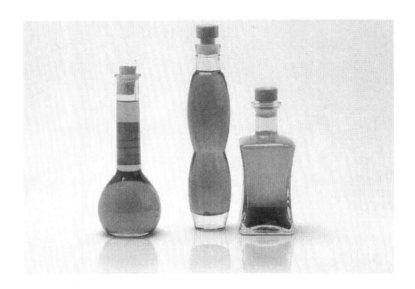

Apple Cider Vinegar has many wonderful uses. No wonder it is considered a miracle compound.
However, because of its high acidic nature it must be used with care. Apple cider vinegar can be considered safe it you are using it in small quantities. It is not recommended that you ingest large amounts.

Evelyn Carmichael

In fact, for safety sake, doctors do not recommend that you take more than eight ounces of ACV in one day [4]. In large amounts, the product has been linked to a drop in potassium levels in the body and suggests that it can cause mineral imbalance. Potassium is important to the body and a lack in this mineral leads to muscle cramps and weakness. Apple cider vinegar interacts with calcium also and this can lead to lower bone density.

If you have diabetes and are considering taking ACV, it is recommended that you consult with your doctor first. Apple cider vinegar is known to reduce blood sugar levels. You may be wondering, so what's the worry, that is your aim. The goal, however, is to maintain blood sugar at a normal level and ACV may be too effective, bringing your levels below normal if used in excess.

Another consideration when taking ACV is that it can interact with some drugs. This can either make you sick or render the drug ineffective for the purpose you are taking it. It important to have a talk with your doctor before you introduce ACV into your daily diet.

Be mindful also that ACV is very acidic and if taken in its natural undiluted state could be too harsh on the gullet when swallowing. You also risk damaging the enamel of your teeth. It is recommended that you dilute it in at least one to three parts water. You could also mix it in your fruit juices or with honey to temper the acidic taste and make it milder for the palate. If you suffer from conditions such as ulcer of the stomach and intestines, it is best not to ingest ACV without consulting your physician.

If you are using ACV on irritated skin as in a sunburn or eczema, you initially may want to apply it directly. However, this might be too harsh and you could get too much of a sting out of it. You would be better off diluting the substance. Pour the diluted substance on a wet wash cloth and rest it over the affected area.

ACV can do wonders for your health, home, and body. Just use it safely, consult with a physician if you have any underlying conditions, and use it in moderation for the most optimal results.

Evelyn Carmichael

REFERENCES

1. Cutler, N. (2012, May 2). Is Apple Cider Vinegar Good for Your Health? Retrieved from: http://www.naturalwellness.com/nwupdate/is-apple-cider-vinegar-good-for-your-health/

2. Gunner, K. (2016). 6 Proven Benefits of Apple Cider Vinegar. Retrieved from: https://authoritynutrition.com/6-proven-health-benefits-of-apple-cider-vinegar/

3. Johnson, B. (2016). The Great Plague. Retrieved from: http://www.historic-uk.com/HistoryUK/HistoryofEngland/The-Great-Plague/

4. Mitchell, L. (2012, August 21). 15 Reasons to Use Apple Cider Vinegar Every Day. Retrieved from: http://www.mindbodygreen.com/0-5875/15-Reasons-to-Use-Apple-Cider-Vinegar-Every-Day.html

Evelyn Carmichael

ABOUT THE AUTHOR

Evelyn Carmichael

Evelyn was in the world of corporate finance before switching her life path after a successful battle with breast cancer. She is a personal life coach, fitness guru, and healthy lifestyle advocate.

Follow Evelyn on Facebook for healthy living tips and information on new releases or at https://www.amazon.com/Evelyn-Carmichael/e/B01MQYHZLC

Evelyn Carmichael

OTHER BOOKS BY EVELYN CARMICHAEL

Evelyn is the author of the Essential Handbook Series.

Her titles include the following:

The Essential Handbook to the Alzheimer's Diet

The Essential Handbook to Superfood Smoothies

The Essential Handbook to Hashimoto's

The Essential Handbook to Hygge

The Essential Handbook to Diabetic Instant Pot Cooking

The Essential Handbook to Gluten Free Instant Pot Cooking

The Essential Handbook to Avocados The Superfood that Reduce Inflammation and lowers blood sugar, blood pressure, and your cholesterol

The Essential Handbook to Reversing Prediabetes and Diabetes: Meal Plans and Recipes to Reduce Your Blood Sugar Levels and Eliminate Diabetes and Prediabetes

Evelyn Carmichael

The Essential Handbook to Turmeric and Ginger: The Anti-Inflammatory Duo that will Change your Life

The Essential Handbook to Coconut Oil: Tips, Recipes, and How to use for weight loss and in your daily life

The Essential Handbook to Apple Cider Vinegar: Tips and Recipes for Weight Loss and Improving your Health, Beauty, & Home

The Art of Keeping Goals

The Essential Handbook for Choosing the Right Diet: A Guide to the Most Popular Diets and if They are Right for You

The Essential Handbook to Natural Living

The Essential Handbook to Essential Oils: Tips and Recipes for Weight Loss, Stress Relief, and Pain Management

Knee Supports: Uses, Exercises, and Benefits

The Essential Handbook for Apple Cider Vinegar

Evelyn Carmichael

AUTHOR NOTE

If you enjoyed this book, found it useful or otherwise then I'd really appreciate it if you would post a short review on Amazon. I do read all the reviews personally so that I can continually write what people are wanting.

Thanks for your support!

Evelyn Carmichael

Made in the USA
Middletown, DE
02 April 2018